Simple Keto Diet Cookbook

for Beginners

Lose weight easily and Live healthy with amazing low carb recipes

By

Ellen Brewer

PART ONE

PART TWO

LOW CARBS KETOGENIC APPETISERS .

PART THREE

LOW CARB SIDE DISH AND SALAD RECIPES

PART FOUR
LOW CARB SAUCE, DRESSINGS AND   CONDIMENT RECIPES

.

PART FIVE

DESSERT RECIPES (LOW CARB)

Copyright©2019

DISCLAIMER

This publication is designed to provide competent and
reliable information regarding the subject matter. However, it is sold with

the understanding that the author is not engaged in rendering professional advice. If an expert assistance is required, the services of a professional should Be Sought.
The author specifically negate any liability that is
incurred from the use or application of the Contents of this material.

Introduction

The ketogenic diet was introduced between 1920s-
30s to help curb seizures in epileptic children.
This diet will force the body to burn fat instead of
carbohydrates, because the carbohydrates in the
food is converted into glucose which is specifically
substantial for charging the brain.
However, the Liver converts fat into fatty acid and

ketone bodies which replaces glucose as
an energy
source.
These ketone bodies leads to drastic
decline in
prevalence of epileptic seizures.
In the 1970s, the ketogenic diet started
gaining
abundant concentration as a promising
weight-loss
strategy due Low-Carb diet trend.
Today, the
ketogenic diet is distinguished for its
extraordinary
high-fat content with moderate protein
intake.
In this cookbook:
• You'll be exposed to varieties of
ketogenic
   Recipes.
• You'll learn how to prepare these
recipes with a step
   By step guide.

• You'll also be exposed to pocket friendly and

Readily available recipes.
And much more!
Without further ado, let's get in the kitchen.

THE KETO BBQs AND RECIPES

Chicken skewers with rosemary buttermilk.

Low carb stuffed zucchini and BBQ chicken.

Hot dog with BBQ bacon cheese.

Avocado salsa diet with grilled salmon.

Skewers of shrimp scampi.

Northern fried chicken recipe.

Onion soup with London broil.

Burgers stuffed with caramelised onion and Brie.

Yogurt sauce with chicken souvlaki.

Shrimp of pesto.

The Barbecue ribs jerk.
1. Chicken Skewers with Rosemary   Buttermilk
Introduction:

Ingredients:
Chicken breast (boneless) (2kg)
Butter milk (One cup),
 Virgin Olive oil (one-third cup)
 Worcestershire sauce (Two tablespoon)
 Valley ranch dressing (one Oz)
Fresh pepper (Half teaspoon)
Minced rosemary (Two sprigs)

How To prepare :
 1. Cut all your chicken into smaller sizes like a cube
 2. Soak for thirty minutes then arrange them properly on a skew
3. Add your marinade and keep in a refrigerator
4. Preheat your grill at a moderate temperature. Dress   and keep chicken meat on it and allow to cook.

5. Cook for twenty minutes and its ready to serve

2.   Low Carb Stuffed Zucchini and BBQ

Introduction :

Ingredients:

Sugar ketchup (one-third cup)
Cider vinegar (one-quarter cup)
Onion powder (One teaspoon)

Yellow mustard (Two teaspoon)

Granulated sugar (Two tablespoon)

Liquid smoke (one-quarter teaspoon)

Mayonnaise (Two tablespoon)
Chopped cilantro (two tablespoon)
Chopped red onion (Two tablespoon)
Raw corn kernels (one-quarter cup)
Cooked chicken (Two cups)
Zucchini (Two)

Shredded Jack cheese (Half cup)

How To prepare

1. Mix the following in a bowl, Whisk the cider vinegar, onion powder, mustard,

sweetener, Mayonnaise, liquid smoke
and ketchup and add the next
ingredient which is corn kernels,
cilantro and red onion and whisk
properly while you add the shredded
chicken.
2. Now you have to heat up the
zucchini
And then season with pepper salt. Heat
for 5 minutes and it becomes soft

3. Now you need to preheat the oven
because we shall be baking out zucchini.
Add an amount of BBQ chicken to this
and baking at 350 degrees heat for
thirty minutes
4. When ready, Serve and enjoy your
meal.
Nutritional information
This recipe has 4 servings and each
Serving contains 27g protein, 17g fat,
6.5g carbs and 290 calories.

3. Hot Dog with BBQ Bacon Cheese

Introduction :

Ingredients:
   Hot dogs (eight)
   Gouda cheese (eight slices)
   Bacon (sixteen slices)
   BBQ sauce (Half cup)
   Tasted hot dog buns (Eight)

Procedure :
 1. Cut and chop the hot dog into bits sizes as desired
 2. Cut two bacon slices and hold your hot dog with it. Ensure that toothpicks are added to it so as to keep things in proper position
 3. Pass the wrapped hot dog in a grill and heat gently until the bacon becomes crisp and you notice a sweat like heat around the wrap.
 4. Serve and enjoy

4. Avocado Salsa Diet with Grilled Salmon

Introduction:

Ingredients:

1. Salmon (two kilogram)
2. Olive oil (one tablespoon)
3. Salt (one teaspoon)
4. Ground cumin (One teaspoon)
5. Paprika powder (one teaspoon)
6. Chilli powder (Half teaspoon)
7. Black pepper (one teaspoon)
8. Sliced avocado (one)
9. Sliced red onion (half)
10. Lime juice (half-cup)
11. Chopped cilantro (two tablespoon)
12. Salt.

How To prepare:

1. Get a bowl and be ready to mix the following ingredients paprika, onion, cumin, chili powder, salt coat   salmon fillet with the seasoning mix and olive oil.

2. Refrigerate for   45 minutes;

Add the following to your juice mix lime juice, cilantro, onion, avocado and salt and allow to cool for some time.

3. Put the salmon in a grill and allow for some minutes to grill. Between 5-7 minutes

4. Sprinkle the recipe with avocado salsa.

5. Serve.

Nutritional information-- This serving contains 21g protein, 19g carbs, 22g fats and 366 calories.

5. Skewers of Shrimp Scampi

Introduction :

Ingredients :
1. Large raw shrimp (One pound)
2. Lemons (3)
3. Kosher salt (Half teaspoon)
4. Black pepper (Half teaspoon)
5. Red pepper flakes(one-eight spoon)

6. Parsley butter with garlic: Butter (Three tablespoon), Minced garlic (Two cloves), Dry white wine (One quarter cup), fresh parsley (One-quarter cup)

How To prepare:

1. Melt the butter by heating in a microwave oven. This is the first step.

2. Pour the white wine in a pan containing the molten butter add your garlic and steam for about three minutes

3. Coat Shrimps with red peppers, salt and black pepper and arrange along a skewer

4. Grill for 5 minutes and you will notice that the colour of shrimp is now pink. Remove from grill.

5. Serve and enjoy.

6. Northern Fried Chicken Recipe

Introduction:

Ingredients :

1. Chicken leg (5kg)

2. Salt (one teaspoon)

3. Garlic powder (one teaspoon)

4. Paprika (one teaspoon)
5. Coconut flour (one cup)
6. Oil.

Procedure :

Get a whole chicken and prepare it for this purpose.

Mix the following ingredients, the pepper, garlic powder, salt, chicken and paprika.

To ensure the spices are evenly distributed, mix with your hands thoroughly.

2. Now you should Refrigerate for 60 minutes.

3. Now we shall add some coconut flour to the chicken to give it a coat.

4. Yes, we can now fry the chicken till it become crisp and the colour becomes golden.

Serve and enjoy

7. Onion Soup with London Broil

Introduction:

Ingredients :

London broils (one and half pounds)
Olive oil (2 tablespoon)
Onion soup seasoning (one-quarter cup)
Dried onion flakes (one-quarter cup)
Onion powder (one teaspoon)
Sea salt (half teaspoon)
Palm sugar (Half teaspoon)

How To prepare:

1. Rub meat with oil and coat with the onion soup mix that we have prepared
2. Using aluminium foil as protective, broil meat on each side.
3. Remove from the heat. Allow some time for it to set.
4. Serve and Enjoy!

8. Burgers Stuffed with Brie

Introduction :

Ingredients :

Mushrooms: - Butter (Two tablespoon) Sliced mushroom Salt

 Burgers: Ground beef (two ibs) Salt (half teaspoon) Ground pepper (half teaspoon)

Brie cheese (4 ounce)

Salt (Half teaspoon)

Olive oil (Two tablespoon)

Sliced onions (one)

How To prepare:

 1. pour some olive oil in a pan, add salt and then your onions. Heat up your onions in medium or moderate heat

 2. Cook for 30 minutes and watch carefully until you notice a change in colour.

 3. mix pepper , salt and beef in a bowl or container using your hands. Scoop and divide from the mix six parts

4. Form nice patties in each portion and put onions and brie
 5. Preheat oven or grill for 130 degrees and cook the portions
 Cook for seven minutes and allow to cool
 6. Cook the mushrooms till it's brown in color and ready to serve
Serve and enjoy

9. Yogurt Sauce with Chicken Souvlaki

Ingredients :

For the yoghurt sauce, you need the following:
 1. Lemon juice (one teaspoon)
 2. Minced garlic (one teaspoon)
 3. Fresh oregano (one teaspoon)
 4. Greek yogurt (Three-quarter cup)
 5. Granulated sugar (half teaspoon).
For the Chicken, you need the following:
 1. Chicken breast (One Kilogram)
 2. Olive oil (three tablespoon)

3. Lemon juice (Three tablespoon)
4. Red wine (One tablespoon)
5. Minced garlic (Four cloves)
6. Kosher salt (Two tablespoon)
7. Black pepper
(one-quarter teaspoon)
8. Dried thyme (Half teaspoon)

How To prepare of Yogurt Sauce

1. After getting the ingredients for the yoghurt, mix them together very well.

2. Stir continuously until you get a consistent mixture and serve with your chicken souvlaki.

How To prepare of Chicken Souvlaki

1. get a bowl and mix the following lemon juice, red wine, olive oil, garlic, salt, oregano, pepper and dried thyme together
in a dish.

2 add chicken and marinade and mix thoroughly, after this, refrigerate for 1 hour

3. put your chicken in a grill and pre-

heating for 5 minutes.

4. Serve and enjoy recipe with yoghurt

10 Shrimp of Pesto

Introduction :

Ingredients :

1. Frozen and fresh shrimp (24 oz).

2. Pesto sauce (Half cup).

How To prepare:

1. Bring your skewers and arrange them. Get shrimp soaked in the water for over half an hour.

2. Using aluminium foil, take shrimp and arrange them properly then coat with pesto sauce

3. Now you will arrange the shrimps that are now coated on the grill

Broil the shrimp for five minutes and flip the other side

4. Serve and enjoy meal

Nutritional information

Each serving contains 38g protein, 0.6g fibre,

508mg sodium, 0.2g sugar, 3g carbohydrates and 36g fats.

11. The Ribs Jerk Barbecue

Introduction:

Ingredients :

1. Pork ribs (one rack)
2. Caribbean jerk seasoning (half cup)

Sauce Ingredients:

Tamari (one quarter cup)
Soya sauce Water (one-quarter)
Fresh ginger (Two tablespoon)
Orange zest (Two tablespoon)
Orange juice (One-quarter cup)
White vinegar (one quarter cup)
Worcestershire sauce (One)
Rice wine vinegar (two tablespoon)
Sugar substitute (Paleo/honey) (Three tablespoon)
Xanthan gum (one teaspoon)

How To prepare:

1. Preheat oven at 330 degrees , coat the ribs and bake at this temperature

2. Mix the following thoroughly ginger, water, soy sauce, White vinegar, Worcestershire , sauce, orange zest, rice wine vinegar and dozen mustard in a bowl and boil for ten minutes

3. Strain your sauce to take away the ginger and orange zest and add sweetener and xanthum gum.

4. The ribs that has now been cooked will be coated with sauce and cooked at 380 degrees

5. Serve and enjoy.

Nutritional information

Serving - 6

Containing 20g fat, 3g carbs and 34g protein and 320 calories.

PART TWO

LOW CARB KETOGENIC APPETISERS AND SNACKS

1. Low Carb Cheese Roll Ups and Salami

Introduction

Ingredients:

1. Chopped banana peppers (seven and half teaspoon)

2. Chopped red pepper (seven and half teaspoon)

3. Cream cheese (one and half ounce)

4. Salami (fifteen slices)

How To prepare:

1. Bring out the sliced salami and sprinkle your pepper and cheese on them

2. Fold the salami into a taco and sprinkle your banana pepper on the five cut slice

3. Attach your toothpick and make them firm

4. Serve and enjoy your meal.

Nutritional information

S ervings 5 and each of the serving contains 2.80 g of protein, 4.50 g fats, 50 calories, 0.62 g carbs and 2.55 g fibres.

2. Jalapeno Poppers

Introduction:

Ingredients :

1. Jalapeno peppers (Ten)
2. Slices of Bacon (Ten)
3. Mini smokies or sausages (Ten)
4. Cream cheese (one cup)
5. Grated Monterey jack (one cup)
6. Chilli powder (one teaspoon)
7. Minced shallots (two)

How To prepare:

1. Take some jalapenos and remove the membrane, now begin to cut them length wise or vertically.

2. Get a bowl or container and begin to mix the following minced shallots, chili powder, Monterey jack and cream cheese

3. Fill the jalapenos with this mixture
wrap your jalapenos with bacon and
allow enough smoke to touch the
cream cheese.
Preheat oven at 225 degrees till your
bacon turns brown.
5. Serve and enjoy

3. Low Carb Mediterranean Eggs Recipe

Introduction

Ingredients:
1. Large eggs (one dozen)
2. Mayonnaise (Half cup)
3. Dizon mustard (one teaspoon)
4. Chopped capers (one tablespoon)
5. Kalamata olives (one tablespoon))
6. Chopped tomatoes (one teaspoon)
7. Olive oil (one tablespoon)
8. Minced basil (Two tablespoon))
9. Caper brine (one teaspoon)
10. Pepper and salt.

How To prepare:

1. Firstly, you need to boil the eggs.
After about 8 minutes, bring it down.
Now allow them to remain in the water
for twenty limits.

2. Half slice all the eggs after removing
from hot water

3. Get a bowl and a fork, smash the
egg yolks very well in a container

4. Now add your mustard,
mayonnaise, capers, sun-dried
tomatoes, basil, olive oil and caper
brine properly in your food processor.

5. Now in the egg yolk, add pepper and
salt and

6. Serve and enjoy.

Nutritional information

Each serving contains 80 calories, 8g
fats and 6g proteins.

4. Low Carb Perfect Guacamole
Introduction

Ingredients:

1. Avocados (Two)
2. Kosher salt (Half teaspoon)

3. Lemon juice (one tablespoon)
4. Chopped cilantro (Two Tablespoon)
5. Minced red Onion (two tablespoon)
6. Minced Serrano chiles (Two)
7. Chopped ripe tomatoes (Two)
8. Black pepper

How To prepare:

1. Dissect your Avocado into 2 equal halves and then scoop out the seed and the flesh using your spoon into a medium sized bowl.

2. Mash your avocado with the fork and then add your lime juice and salt. (The essence of the lime juice is to provide a balance to the alkalinity and prevent the avocado from changing into a brown colour)

3. Put your black pepper, cilantro, chopped onion and chiles and then use

a plastic wrap to cover the guacamole surface and refrigerate.

4. Serve while cool and enjoy your guacamole.

5. Barbecue Shrimp Wrapped with Keto Bacon

Introduction:

This recipe is fully loaded with amazing flavours which will provide good and

Enriching diets that will leave you Begging for more of these delicious diets.

Ingredients:

1. Bacon (Eight)
2. Shrimp (Sixteen)
3. Sauce (Two tablespoon)
4. Water (Half cup)
5. Chipotle powder (Half teaspoon)
6. Lime juice (Two teaspoon)
7. Granulated sugar (One teaspoon)

How To prepare:

1. In a heat-proved pan, boil the bacon till it becomes pretty brownish or for 5 minutes.

2. Mix your sweetener, lime juice, powder, water and the sauce in a medium pan.

3. Mix your prepared sauce with the precooked bacon and heat gently for about 5 minutes.

4. Dissect the bacon into about sixteen pieces after removing it from the sauce.

5. Inside your sauce, put the shrimp and allow for one minute.

6. Wrap bacon to each piece of the shrimp after removal from the sauce and then skewer.

7. Grill the skewers for a minute on each side while ensuring it didn't stick onto the pan.

8. Serve while warm and enjoy.

You can put more lime wedges if you want it that way.

6. Hot Dog Keto Recipe

Introduction:

Ingredients:

1. Keto Buns (Half recipe)
2. Sausages
3. Egg yolk (one)
4. Sesame or sunflower seeds (Two tablespoon)
5. Course salt (Half teaspoon)
6. Optional – Dijon mustard.

How To prepare:

1. Get a good mixer and make a hot dog dough in it
2. Refrigerate the wrapped foil containing the

   dough for a period of 40 minutes. Divide the

   dough into five equal parts.

3. Using wet hands, cut each dough size into fifteen
     parts or pieces.
4. Preheat an oven at 350degrees so that we can
     bake.

5. Using a baking sheet, spread this on a flat
     surface, pour an ample amount of dough and
     spread with a mixture of egg yolk and seeds then
     repeat the same process for the rest of the
     dough.
6. Set on the oven for fifty minutes and heat
   Until it becomes golden brown.
7. After baking, put it into your serving plate
     and enjoy with BBQ sauce or ketch up.

Nutritional information

The hot dog keto recipe has 6 servings and each contain 9.6g fibres, 20g protein, 25g fats and 350 calories

7. Low Carb Pups And Dogs Recipes:

Introduction :

Ingredients:
1. Honeyville Almond flour (one cup).
2. Coconut flour (Three tablespoon)
3. Corn meal (Three tablespoon)
4. Salt (one-quarter teaspoon)
5. Erythritol (one tablespoon)
6. Baking powder (one quarter teaspoon)
7. Xanthan gum (one-quarter teaspoon)
8. Eggs (Three)
9. Oil (Two teaspoon)

10. Coconut milk(one-third cup)

11. Coconut flour (one tablespoon)

How To prepare:

1. Get a chop stick, put them inside the hot dog

2. Preheat your oil, get a bowl and whisk all the corn dog ingredients in this bowl then set it aside

3. Repeat the same process with the wet ingredients

4. Sprinkle the coconut on the body after drying it with a paper towel
Make sure you coat the body properly

5. Bake the corn dog in the oil for some minutes and flip the other side after a brown color is reach.

6. Keep them aside and repeat the baking process for the remainder.

7. If you have any left then add more corn dog batter into the oil and fry until it becomes brown

Nutritional information

Each serving contains 150 calories, 15g
fat, 6g carbohydrates, 2g fibre and 3g protein.

LOW CARB SIDE DISH AND SALAD

RECIPES

- **Potato salad low carb recipe**
- **Low carb keto corn bread**
- **Low carb cauliflower salad and shrimp**
- **Pine nuts and feta with grilled zucchini.**
- **Flow carb Cobb salad**
- **Broccoli salad**
- **Balsamic reduction with salad of tomato mozzarella.**
- **Pecan vinaigrette (toasted and grilled asparagus)**
- **Smith apple slaw.**

1. Potato Salad Low Carb Recipe

Introduction:

Ingredients:

Vegetable Spices:

1. Apple cider vinegar (one tablespoon)
2. Black peppercorns (one teaspoon)
3. Bay leaves (Two)
4. Salt (Half teaspoon)

Salad and Dressing Ingredients:

1. Turnip (one medium)
2. Cucumbers (six)
3. Large eggs (six)
4. Onion (one)
5. Celery stalk (sliced)(one)
6. Mayonnaise (Three-quarter cup)

7. Dijon mustard (1 teaspoon)

8. Chopped parsley (Two tablespoon)
9. Vinegar (Two tablespoon)
10. Celery seeds (one teaspoon)
11. Salt (half teaspoon)
12. Black pepper.

How To prepare:

1. Boil the eggs properly and remove them when they are well cooked after 10 minutes. Next you put them inside cold water. Do not allow them to crack

2. Now is the time you prepare your vegetables. Peel the following;   turnip, celeries and rutabaga very well when you are done, cut them into smaller chunks and pour them into a bowl.
3. Add your vinegar, bay leaves, salt and peppercorns.
 4. Boil for some time until they are tender looking then set aside and allow to cool
 5. Get some onions and dice them add them to your bowl mixture
 6. Remove the eggs from the cold water and peel them carefully removing the shells
 6. Cut the eggs into small pieces and add them to the bowl containing the mixture.

7. Mix the Dijon, celery stalks, all other vegetables together and add salt and pepper to taste then mix thoroughly. keep in the Refrigerator for 24 hours and then
Serve for the family.

2. Low Carb Keto Corn Bread

Introduction:

Ingredients:
Dry Ingredients:
Bacon grease (one tablespoon)
Pork rinds (one-third cup)
Parmesan cheese (Three tablespoon)
Whey protein (Two tablespoon)
Baking powder (Half teaspoon)
Kosher salt (one pinch)

Wet Ingredients:
1. Sour cream (Two tablespoon)
2. Egg (one)
3. Extract of Amoretti popcorn (one-eight teaspoon)
4. Apple cider vinegar (one teaspoon)

How To prepare:

1. Heat the corn bread for five minutes in an oven that have been preheated for 400 degrees Fahrenheit , then add the bacon grease

2. Get q separate bowl and repeat the same process for the wet ingredients. And mix them

3. Now we shall mix both our dry ingredients and our wet ingredient in the same bowl. Suing a spatula, mix them thoroughly.

4. Preheat the oven at 400 degree Fahrenheit and begin to bake your mixture

5. When done, you should serve and enjoy

Nutritional information

Each serving of this recipe contains 15g

protein, 18g fats, 210 calories, 3g carbohydrates, 2g carbs and 0g fibers.

3. Low Carb Cauliflower Salad And Shrimp
 Introduction:

 Ingredients:

1. Cauliflower (one head)
2. Raw shrimp (one)
3. Olive oil (one tablespoon)
4. Cucumbers (Two)
5. Fresh dill (three tablespoon)
6. Olive oil (one-quarter)
7. Lemon Juice (one-quarter cup)
8. Lemon zest (two tablespoon)
9. Pepper and salt.

How To prepare:

1. Get ready the shrimps. Peel the hard cover of the shrimps to get the tender skin. Sprinkle with pepper and salt and fry with the olive oil.

For eight minutes at 350 degrees until it becomes brown

2. Cut the cauliflower into small bits and microwave for 5 minutes. When it's done, allow to cool.

3. Cut the cucumbers into small bits and pieces. Don't forget that the shrimps should also be cut lengthwise.

4. Mix the following cucumber, cauliflower and shrimp in a bowl and put the chopped dill and lemon zest.

5. Coat the mixture with lemon juice and olive oil. Then after that, you add your seasoning with pepper

7. Serve and enjoy your meal.

Nutritional information

Each serving contains 220 calories, 13g fats, 5g carbohydrates and 18g protein.

4. Pine Nuts And Feta With Grilled Zucchini

Introduction:

Ingredients :

1. Zucchini (Four pieces)
3. Olive oil (one tablespoon)
4. Oregano (one and half tablespoon)

5. Black pepper

6. Kosher salt
7. Lemon zest
8. Goat cheese (Three ounces)
9. Pine nuts (one quarter cup)
10. Parsley leaves (one-quarter cup)

How To prepare:

1. Pre-heat your oven or grill. Cut the zucchini into strips as intended for use

2. Mix the zucchini in a bowl with kosher salt then add some olive oil to the mix. This will serve as a coat, then add some black pepper.

3. Grill the mixture for some minutes and add lemon on it.

4. To the softened zucchini, add your pine nuts, goat cheese, parsley leaves and lemon zest.

5. Bring to dining room table and serve.

5. Sesame Ginger with Noodles Of Broccoli Stem
Introduction:

.

Ingredients :

1. Broccoli stems (4)
2. Sesame oil (Two tablespoon
3. Soy sauce (one tablespoon)
4. Minced garlic (two cloves)
5. Grated ginger (one teaspoon)
6. Salt (half teaspoon)
7. Flakes of red pepper (one-quarter)
8. Sesame seeds (two tablespoon)

How To prepare:

1. Get some broccoli stem. Wash them carefully. We are going to use our Spiraliser to form some strips with it.
2. Mix the following in a separate bowl; sesame oil, apple cider vinegar, soy sauce, salt, ginger, flakes of red pepper and pepper.
3. Pour the above mix into the broccoli noodles
4. Serve and enjoy!

Nutritional information
This recipe has four servings and each serving contain 10.2g fats, 10.04g fibres,
4.05g protein and 7.62g carbs.

Low carb salad diets

Introduction

Ingredients:
1. Arugula (Two and half ounces)
2. Egg (one)
3. Grilled chicken (Two ounces)

4. Bacon (Two and half)
5. Green onion (Half ounce)
6. Red pepper (One ounce)
7. Ripe avocado (one and half ounces)
8. Garlic (Three tablespoons)

How To prepare:

1. Boil the eggs and after this, allow them to cool in a bowl in cold water. They should be soaked in it.

2. Now it is time for our bacon to be cooked. Cook the bacon and allow it to become crisp.

3. Add the following ingredients after slicing them, red pepper, green onion, avocado, egg and the blue cheese crumbled

4. Arrange as desired. Scoop out each ingredient
and place carefully on the plate. If you love aesthetics, you will know which should come first.

5. Serve and enjoy

Nutritional information

This recipe has one serving and it contains 570 calories, 48g fats, 9g carbohydrates, 5g fibre and 35g protein.

6. Broccoli Salad

Introduction:

Ingredients:
1.   Broccoli (six cups)
2. Chopped onions (one-quarter)
3. Mayonnaise (a cup)
4. Chopped almonds (Half cup)
5. Red vinegar (Two tablespoon)
 6. Bacon (Eight slices)
7. Pepper and salt.

How to prepare:
1. Get a bowl and mix some bacon with chopped onions in them
2. In another different bowl, add the following ingredients together your vinegar, mayonnaise,
pepper and salt

3. Now sprinkle the mixture on your broccoli and make sure you have an even coat.

4. keep in the refrigerator, Serve when ready and enjoy.

8. Balsamic Reduction with Salad Of Tomato Mozzarella

Introduction :

Ingredients:

1. Sliced tomatoes (Five)

2. Fresh sliced mozzarella cheese (Sixteen ounce)

3. Basil leaves

4. Olive oil

5. Black pepper and sea salt.

6. Balsamic vinegar (two cups) for Balsamic reduction.

How to prepare:

1. Arrange in order the following ingredients, basil, mozzarella and

tomato slices. Let it form two simple rows each

 2. Add some olive oil upon the salad (sprinkle them) after this, also sprinkle the balsamic reduction

 3. Add black pepper and salt.
For the reduction, cook balsamic vinegar for one hour until it becomes a black gaze
Allow to cool and serve it with salad

9.   Pecan Vinaigrette (Toasted) and Grilled Asparagus
Introduction

Ingredients :
1. Trimmed asparagus stalks (one)
2. Olive oil (One teaspoon)
3. Kosher salt.
Vinaigrette Ingredients:
1. Sriracha sauce (one teaspoon)
2. Soy sauce (Two teaspoon)

3. Wine vinegar.
4. Granulated sugar (one sugar)
5. Lime juice (one juice)
6. Toasted pecans (two tablespoon)
7. Grape-seed, avocado or olive oil(1/4) cup.

How To prepare:

Get some asparagus stalks and wash them properly. Get them ready for grilling.

Grill the asparagus and add salt and pepper.

In a separate bowl, mix all other ingredients together.

3. Add some vinaigrette on this asparagus and its ready to be served

Nutritional information

This recipe serving contains 18g fat, 170 calories, 4.03g carbs and 5g protein.

Smith Apple Slaw

Introduction:

Ingredients.

1. Lemon juice (one tablespoon)
2. Red cabbage (eight cups)
3. Chopped mint (one-quarter cup)
4. Avocado oil (one-quarter cup)
5. Vinegar (apple cider) (two tablespoon)
6. Granulated sugar/substitute (one tablespoon)

7. Chopped smith apples (Two cups)

How To prepare:

1. Get three separate bowls and do this. Cut the apples and mix with lemon juice. In another bowl, mix your mint, cabbage and apple and in the third bowl; mix the sweetener, vinegar and oil together.

2. Add the dressing on the Shaw whisk to coat very well. Refrigerate and serve while fresh.

It can be stored for five days in the refrigerator but best eaten under two hours of refrigeration.

Nutritional information

This recipe contains 7g fats, 85 calories, 6g carbs and

2g protein.

LOW CARB SAUCE, DRESSINGS AND CONDIMENT RECIPES.

- Chocolate Barbecue sauce.
- Mango Barbecue sauce with smoky tomato.
- Vinaigrette herb with garlic.
- Pesto of green radish
- Barbecue sugar-free sauce.
- Recipe of pesto
- Gorgonzola butter with ribeye steak
- 30 seconds Caesar dressing.

1. Chocolate Barbecue Sauce
Introduction:

Ingredients :
  1. Ketchup (one cup)
  2. Crushed garlic (two cloves)
  3. Coconut oil (Two tablespoon)
  4. Paprika (Two teaspoon)
  5. Chilli powder (one teaspoon)
  6. Cocoa powder (Two tablespoon)

7. Apple Cider vinegar (Two tablespoon).
  8. Coconut aminos (Two tablespoon)
  9. Erythritol (Two tablespoon)
  10. Stevia extract (10 drops)
  11. Black pepper and salt.

How To prepare:
  1. Measure all the ingredients as species and cut your garlic. While doing this, get a sauce pan ready.
  2. Place the ingredients (butter ketchup, garlic, vinegar, coconut amino, cocoa powder, smoked salt, chilli powder, smoked salt, chilli

powder, stevia, pepper and erythritol)
 into a saucepan and mix properly.
 3. Cook with a low temperature oven
for ten minutes

4. Remove from oven and refrigerate.
5. Serve and enjoy as you wish

2.Tomato and Mango Sauce Barbecue
Introduction:

Ingredients:

1. Tomato puree (Two cups)
2. White vinegar (Half cup)
3. Dijon mustard (one-quarter cup)
4. Ketchup (one-quarter cup)
5. Sugar substitute (one-quarter cup)
6. Liquid smoke (one tablespoon)
7. Apple cider vinegar (one tablespoon)
8. Fish sauce (one teaspoon)
9. Lemon juice (two tablespoon)

10. Dehydrated onions (two tablespoon)

11. Ground coriander (one tablespoon)

12. Celery salt (half teaspoon)

13. Cayenne pepper (one teaspoon)

14. Smoked paprika (one teaspoon)

15. Garlic powder (one tablespoon)

16. Cinnamon (half teaspoon)

17. Allspice (half teaspoon)

18. Cardamom powder (half teaspoon)

19. Ground ginger (one teaspoon)

20. Ground cloves (half teaspoon)

21. Mango syrup (one tablespoon)- Optional

How To prepare:

In a pan mix all the above mentioned ingredients. It may seem much but that's how we prepare this.
Steam them for sometime

2. Add your salt to taste.

3. Serve this along with your main dish and enjoy.

3. Vinaigrette Herb with Garlic

Introduction:

Ingredients :
1. Olive oil (half cup)
2. Champagne vinegar (one-quarter cup)
3. Powdered erythritol (one teaspoon)

4. Lemon zest (one teaspoon)
5. Water (two tablespoon)
6. Salt.

How To prepare:

Firstly, we need to measure all our ingredients into a dish and then mix them properly and pour into a blender.

Blend all ingredient until evenly smooth.

Serve and enjoy.

4. Pesto Of Green Radish
Introduction

Ingredients:

1. Radish green (three cups)
2. Garlic (two cloves)
3. Pine nuts (one- quarter cup)
4. Parmesan cheese (one cup)
5. Olive oil (one-quarter cup)
6. Pepper and Kosher salt.

How To prepare:

Chop the necessary ingredients and mix them up with others in a bowl. Gather them all and pour into food processor container and blend properly to get a uniform mixture.

3. Add pepper and salt to the mixture before you refrigerate.

5. Sugar-Free Barbecue Sauce
Introduction :

Ingredients :
1. Tomato sauce (Fifteen Oz)
2. Onion powder (one tablespoon)
3. Tomato paste (Six Oz)
4. Salt (one tablespoon

5. Garlic powder (one tablespoon)
6. Yellow mustard (One and half tablespoon).
7. Erythritol (two tablespoon)
8. Vinegar (one quarter cup)
9. Molasses (one tablespoon)
10. Liquid smoke (one teaspoon)

How To prepare:

Get all the listed ingredients and begin preparing them.
Get a bowl and mix them in it.
Transfer to a cooking pan and cook for some
time until you notice the bubbles. This should be
about fifteen minutes.
Remove from the oven and allow to cool

2. Serve immediately or put in the refrigerator.

It's optional to add the molasses. It spices things up when you do.

6. Recipe of Pesto

Introduction :

Ingredients :

1. Washed basil leaves (one cup)
2. Romano cheese or grated parmesan (one-quarter)
3. Olive oil (one-quarter cup)
4. Pine nuts (one-quarter)
5. Chopped garlic (three cloves)
6. Kosher salt (one-quarter teaspoon)
7. Black pepper. (one-quarter teaspoon)

How To prepare:

1. Mix all food ingredients in the food processors bowl.
2. Keep them in the refrigerator and use when needed

7. Gorgonzola Butter With Ribeye Steak

Introduction:

Ingredients :
1. Ribeye steaks
2. Softened butter (Half cup)
3. Gorgonzola cheese (Two oz)
4. Parsley, chopped (one-quarter cup).
5. Crushed garlic (one clove)
6. Pepper and salt.

How To prepare:

Preheat your oven at 350 degrees and get a pan.

Heat your riyeks steaks gently and add salt and pepper to the sides

Pour some gorgonzola butter (chilled one) and allow for five minutes and serve.

To prepare your Gorgonzola butter: Mix

This butter is made by adding garlic and palsy to gondola butter in a food processor and mix.

8.   30 Seconds Caesar Dressing

Introduction:

Ingredients:
1. Pasteurised egg (one)

2. Olive oil (one cup)
3. Parmingiano Reggiano cheese (one-quarter cup)

4. Smashed garlic (one clove)
5. Lemon juice (four tablespoon)
6. Dijon mustard (one and half teaspoon)
7. Black pepper (half teaspoon)
8. Salt (half teaspoon)
9. Anchovy paste (one and half teaspoon).

How To prepare:

1. Leave your egg and oil at room temperature and mix another ingredients in a jar.

2. Get your blender and blend everything thing until they are emulsified. Taste and add any needed seasoning as desired.Refrigerate, serve and enjoy.

Note : pasteurised eggs are used to minimise the effect of bacteria when raw eggs are used

DESSERT RECIPES (LOW CARB)

- Lemon bar dessert
- Coconut fudge (white chocolate)
- Cupcake floats of root beer.
- Cake of strawberry mug

1. Lemon Bar Dessert

Introduction :

Ingredients :

Crust Ingredients:
1. Butter (six tablespoon)

2. Almond flour (two cups)
3. Sugar substitute (one-third cup)
4. Lemon zest (fresh) (one tablespoon)

Filling Ingredients:
1. Butter (half cup)
2. Sugar substitute (e.g. swerve) (half cup)
3. Lemon juice (half cup)
4. Lemon zest (one-quarter cup)
5. Yolks (six egg)
6. Xanthan gum (half teaspoon)
7. Gelatine (two tablespoon).

How To prepare:
For Your Crust:
1. Melt your butter and add sweetener, almond flour, lemon zest and mix properly till evenly mixed. Cook at 350 degree Fahrenheit for 10 minutes. Allow to cool.

For The Filling:

1. In a pan, add butter and heat in the oven. After it melts, add your lemon zest, lemon juice and sweetener.
Mix very well and add your egg yolk and heat gently. Add the gelatine and xanthan gum till all is dissolved
2. Sprinkle the filings for fifteen minutes at a temperature of 350 degree Fahrenheit. Pour away the top swerve if you desire. Serve and enjoy

2. Coconut Fudge (White Chocolate)
Introduction

. **Ingredients:**
1. Cacao butter (four ounces)
2. Coconut milk (one can)
3. Coconut oil (half cup)

4. Coconut butter (one cup)

5. Vanilla protein powder (half cup)

6. Vanilla extract (one teaspoon)

7. Coconut liquid stevia
(one teaspoon)

8. Salt (pinch).

How To prepare:

1. Melt your cocoa butter under a pan under a moderate heat.

2. Add your coconut oil, coconut milk and coconut butter and mix with a spoon continuously

3. Now it is time to bring it down and add stevia, vanilla extract, protein powder and salt.

4. Get some parchment paper and pour the mixture in it. Get it ready for the refrigerator

5. Refrigerate and serve when ready to eat.

3. Cupcakes Floats Of Root Beer

Introduction:

Ingredients:
1. Cacao powder (one-quarter cup)
2. Almond flour (two cups)
3. Whey protein (unflavoured) (one-third cup)
4. Baking powder (two teaspoon)
5. Baking soda (half teaspoon)
6. Xanthan gum (half teaspoon)
7. Salt (one-quarter teaspoon)
8. Butter (five tablespoon)
9. Sweetener (one-third cup)
10. Eggs (two)
11. Extract of root beer (two teaspoon)
12. Stevia extract (one-quarter teaspoon)

Frost Ingredients:
1. Whipping cream (one cup)
2. Swerve sweetener (one-third cup)

3. Extract of vanilla (half teaspoon)

How To prepare:

Firstly, we need to prepare the cupcakes:

1. Pre-heat the oven to 330 degree Fahrenheit. And begin to place your paper liners on the muffin pan

2. Mix the following in a bowl cocoa powder, almond flour, whey protein, baking soda, xanthan gum, and salt.

3. In a medium dish, put the erythritol and butter. Beat till it becomes creamy. Put the extract of root beer, eggs and extract of stevia.

4. Put your almond flour and mix very well and pour the well-mixed compositions into the muffin cups. Bake for thirty minutes and then allow cooling in your pan.

To prepare your frost:

1. Mix your vanilla extract, erythritol (powdered) and cream in a medium dish and beat to get a perfect mixture.

2. Spoon or pipe into your cupcakes.

This dessert has twelve servings and each has about 25g fats, 270 calories,
80g protein, 3g fiber and 4g carbs.

4. Strawberry Mug Cake
Introduction :

.

Ingredients:
For Your Cakes:
1. Butter (two tablespoon)
2. Sugar substitute (two tablespoon)
3. Almond flour (one-quarter cup)
4. Coconut flour (one tablespoon)
5. Egg (one)
6. Strawberries (one-quarter cup)
7. Baking powder (half teaspoon)
8. Vanilla extract (half teaspoon)
For Strawberry Cream:
1. Whipping cream (half cup)

2. Strawberries (two tablespoon)
3. Sugar substitute (one tablespoon.

How To prepare:

For Cake:

  1. Melt all the butter in a frying pan and add all ingredient for mixing

  2. Divide your barter and cook them for few

minutes. Now preheat the oven at 380 degrees and cook all ingredients for some time until its ready to be served.

Conclusion

This brings us to the end of this exercise. I sincerely

hope the recipes and method of application you've

Learned here will help you to achieve the keto lifestyle you desire.

The opportunities for weight-loss and staying healthy are endless, and you're indeed

poised to participate in this development if you

implement the use of the aforementioned recipes

and procedures.